Look Younger

Women's Handbook to Looking Young and Staying Young

Jenna Patterson

Table of Contents

Introduction

Getting older doesn't have to mean *looking* older as well. Thanks to modern science, we now have a much better understanding of how the aging process works and how we can slow down or even reverse the symptoms of aging.

There are a lot of methods out there for making yourself look younger. Unfortunately, many of the products available don't actually work. Expensive miracle creams promising to eliminate wrinkles over night end up making no difference whatsoever. Even more expensive surgeries will work for awhile but eventually the aging process catches up to you.

But that's not the end of the story. Thanks to all the research on how the body ages, you can take control of your appearance and watch the years melt away, all without spending thousands of dollars on surgeries or expensive anti aging products.

With this book, you have a comprehensive guide on how to look younger and fight the aging process. These are proven strategies that will actually work and these are all things you can do without having to stretch your budget.

All of these strategies will be effective no matter what age you are right now. It's never too early or too late to start fighting the aging process and keeping yourself younger. By following the guidelines given in these chapters, you could take decades off your appearance and keep them off.

Before you can do that, you need to have a basic understanding of exactly what causes aging. Getting older does not necessarily have to mean getting wrinkled and weak as well. By understanding what causes the physical signs of aging, you will know how to combat them so that you can grow older while still maintaining a strong, youthful body and mind. Chapter 1 of this book will go over the 7 factors that contribute to the physical signs of aging.

After you understand how aging works, you will learn about:

- foods you should avoid because they speed up the aging process
- foods you should be eating more often because the slow down or reverse the aging process
- how exercising regularly can make you look younger
- different types of exercises and what they do for the body
- sample workout plans and extra tips for keeping up with a workout routine
- recipes for home remedies such as facial masks and skin treatments that can help smooth out wrinkles and revitalize your skin, and;
- fashion tips for dressing yourself to look younger

With all this information, you can fight the aging process from the inside out. You will be able to reverse aging at the cellular level as well as update your external appearance and habits to match the new, younger you!

Chapter 1: The 7 Causes of Aging

The first step to looking younger is knowing what the major causes of aging are. With this information, you will be able to tell exactly how anti-aging techniques work. More importantly, you'll be able to tell the difference between anti-aging methods that work and those that won't work.

There are lots of products out there that promise to make you look younger but many of them don't contain any proven ingredients that actually work to combat these seven causes of aging. This is why it's important to know what causes aging and whether or not a certain product actually fights against any of these things.

Another reason it is important to know the causes of aging is so that you can more effectively combat the aging process. Make up and plastic surgery can only go so far in erasing the signs of age. If you truly want to look younger, you have to *make* yourself younger at the cellular level. This sounds a lot harder than it actually is. Chapters 2 and 3 will provide you with practical ways to fight aging at the cellular level.

Shrinking Tissues and Cell Loss

As your cells age, they will reproduce themselves through cell division in order to create newer, younger cells. When we start to get older, this process of cell reproduction starts to happen at a slower rate and cells start to die off without reproducing themselves. This means that cells get lost at a faster rate than they can be reproduced.

Cell loss leads to shrinking tissues and weaker muscles. Your skin is less firm because there is less tissue to support it. Your bones and muscles also become more brittle. To combat this factor of aging, you need to stimulate cell growth. This is usually done through exercise. You will learn about anti-aging exercises in chapter 3.

Cell Mutations

Another cause of aging is cell mutation. Each time a cell divides itself into two newer cells; there is a potential risk for mutation. Mutations are not necessarily a bad thing and usually, mutations are not noticeable at all.

However, these mutations can become cancerous in certain circumstances and they can also affect how old you appear. There is not sure fire way to prevent cell mutation since it is a completely random process. What you can do, though, is ensure that your cells are healthy. Healthy cells are better able to produce perfect copies of themselves during the cell division process. To keep your cells healthy requires a combination of nutritious food and exercise.

Mitochondrial Mutations

Mitochondria are the cells that play the biggest role in producing energy. They also regulate the entire cycle of a cell's life, including growth. Despite being so essential, they are unfortunately extremely prone to mutation and degradation. As the mitochondria degrade, your cells lose their key source of energy as well as the instructions for growth (which means the cells themselves are at a higher risk for mutation as well).

One of the main reasons that mitochondria begin to degrade or mutate is because they are often exposed to toxins in the body. They are less protected than other cells so these toxins are more dangerous for them. So to prevent mitochondrial mutations, you need to eat a diet rich in antioxidants. You will learn more about antioxidant rich foods in the next chapter.

Zombie Cells

While most cells undergo cell division to split into two new cells, there are some cells that are unable to divide for various reasons. Typically, these are either fat cells or immune system cells. Normally, the body eliminates cells that can no longer die by sending a signal to the cell to kill itself.

However, the cells don't always respond to this signal and will linger in your body, unable to reproduce and unable to die off. When you accumulate too many of these "zombie" cells, it causes visible signs of aging like tissue deterioration. It also makes you more vulnerable to infections.

The best way to fight aging caused by zombie cells is through the combination of a good diet and exercise which will decrease the amount of fat cells in your body and strengthen your immune system. Because fat cells and immune system cells are at the highest risk for becoming zombie cells, this will help decrease that risk.

AGEs and Other Crosslinks

AGE stands for "Advanced Glycation End products." AGEs are a kind of chemical bond or "crosslink." There are multiple kinds of crosslinks but AGEs play the biggest role in the aging process. Crosslinks occur when two proteins bond together. This doesn't sound harmful but when it happens, the proteins becomes stiff and aren't able to move flexibly.

The lack of flexibility causes tissues to become less elastic. This can wreak havoc all over the body. Your blood vessels will become hard, your skin will begin to sag, and your circulation becomes poor. All of these contribute to a body that looks and feels old.

AGEs are produced in your body itself but you also consume them in the foods you eat. In chapter 2, you will learn about foods that are high in AGEs so that you can avoid eating them. You can prevent your body from producing them by eating healthy and exercising.

Build Up Outside Cells

Throughout our lives, we put a lot of stuff into our bodies. We eat food, we breathe in air, we put on lotion that is absorbed into the skin. When we are younger, it is easier for our body to regularly clean out the buildup of excess junk that gets into our bodies and even into our blood streams. But when we get older, our systems start to slow down and the junk material just stays in our bodies.

Plaque buildup in our brain causes Alzheimer's and other mental illnesses. Cholesterol and toxins in the blood slow down circulation and give our skin that grey, wrinkled look. The main systems responsible for clearing out this excess junk are your immune system and your digestive system.

So to prevent excessive build up, you need to eat a healthy diet high in fiber so that your digestive system can continue functioning at full capacity. You also need to eat plenty of immune boosting foods so that your immune system stays strong and can continue clearing out the junk from your blood stream.

Build Up Inside Cells

Just as junk can build up in your blood and throughout your body; it also starts to build up *inside* your cells. Certain proteins and other molecules that usually would get destroyed get trapped inside cells and linger there forever.

This becomes a huge problem in the cells that do not reproduce themselves. When they become too filled with junk, they stop working properly. This causes liver spots on the skin. It can also cause blindness and many other problems.

Fighting build up inside the cells begins with building healthy cells. You need to give your body all the nutrients it needs so that it can feed the cells and keep them strong enough to break down and flush out the junk before it builds up.

Chapter 2: The Age Defying Diet

One of the best ways to combat the aging process is to eat a healthy diet that revitalizes and invigorates your body rather than slowing it down. Eating an age defying diet requires two major steps. First, you have to cut out the biggest offenders that cause the most damage to your skin and appearance. Second, you have to add in the super foods that help slow and even reverse the aging process.

So let's first take a look at the worst offenders and learn how your current diet might actually be working against you:

The Foods That Are Causing You to Age Faster

1. **Anything Deep Fried:** deep fried foods are not only unhealthy in general but terrible for your skin. The process of deep frying foods is a chemical process that destroys the majority of the nutrients and

creates AGEs (Advanced Glycation End products). AGEs are the elasticity killing crosslinks that you read about in chapter one. Any food that is exposed to extremely high heat (as in frying, grilling, or broiling) end up with a load of AGEs that will harm your cells and make your skin sag more quickly.

2. **Refined Sugar:** many studies have come out recently which confirm that refined sugar is a major cause of accelerated aging. In fact, some argue that of all the damaging foods out there, refined sugar causes the most harm. While it doesn't contain AGEs itself, it actually creates them inside your body. As you read, AGEs made inside the body contribute more directly to aging than the ones that you consume in your diet. Beyond that, they also increase the levels of insulin and leptin in your body while *decreasing* your body's ability to process these hormones. This causes an excess of these two hormones which causes premature aging of the skin as well as the organs inside the body. It is also linked to heart disease and

obesity. So, if you decide to give up just one of the 5 things mentioned on this list, choose refined sugar.

3. **Processed Meat:** processed meats like lunch meat, hot dogs or bacon use nitrites to decrease the risk of botulism. However, these nitrites are carcinogenic (i.e. – they increase your risk for cancer). They have also been found to possibly cause infertility in women. Aside from their many health risks, they also speed up the aging process because they eat away the DNA telomeres. DNA telomeres are a sort of protective coating on DNA strands that prevent the DNA from deteriorating. Without this telomere coating, DNA has no protection and will begin to deteriorate and break apart. This will lead to premature aging of your muscles, organs, and skin.

4. **Fatty Meat:** meats like lamb, beef, pork, and sausage are high in fat. While fat is not necessarily bad for you, a diet high in fatty meats can cause premature aging. This is because our digestive systems are not actually meant to process so much animal fat or

animal flesh. It is much easier to digest plant foods and lean meat (fish, poultry, and so on). If you eat too many fatty meats, your system will get backed up. Your metabolism will slow down and you will absorb fewer nutrients. As the fatty meats sit in your system for a long period of time (because they take so long to digest fully), they can actually begin to rot *before* you can fully digest them. Rotting releases a lot of toxins into your body that can cause serious problems like colon cancer but also cause physical deterioration to your skin and muscles. So, while you don't have to cut out fatty meats entirely, you should try to keep it down to once a week.

5. **Alcohol:** drinking an excessive amount of alcohol is unhealthy for a lot of reasons. You are probably already aware of many of the health risks of drinking too much alcohol. But it also plays a huge role in aging. Not only does it cause premature aging but it causes *exaggerated* aging. That is, even if you are at an age where it is natural for you to have some

wrinkles; alcohol will cause you to have even more wrinkles than you would normally have.

Super Foods to Fight the Aging Process

1. **Olive Oil:** eating more olive oil is one of the most incredible things you can do for your skin. Not only will the oil itself keep your skin hydrated and elastic (rather than dry and sagging) but the high vitamin E content will rejuvenate your skin at the cellular level; giving you a fresh, healthy glow. Olive oil will prevent new wrinkles from appearing *and* reduce the wrinkles that are already there. It keeps your skin soft to the touch but also firm and resilient against wrinkling. It is also hypoallergenic so it is safe for everyone to use. You can also use it as a topical skin treatment (you will learn more about this later on in this book). Try to eat at least 2 tablespoons of olive oil per day. You don't have to just eat it plain. You can add it to a salad dressing or even toss a tablespoon into your breakfast smoothie.

2. **Yogurt:** yogurt may not be the first thing you think of when you see the phrase "super food" but it is actually a powerful (and tasty) food. It is high in protein and calcium but low in sugar (if you get the plain kind and add your own fruits and sweeteners). Not only that, it is high in probiotics and healthy bacteria that your digestive system depends on in order to properly break down food and absorb nutrients. It will reduce your risk for age related illnesses and help your body absorb all the nutrients it can from the other healthy foods you eat. This makes plain (*full* fat) yogurt an excellent base that you can dress up however you like with healthy fruits, nuts, herbs or veggies. You can make it a sweet treat as it is most commonly eaten in the US or you can make a savory yogurt dish (like Tzatziki, a popular Greek sauce made of yogurt and used on meat or as a veggie dip).

3. **Fish:** fish is one of the most amazingly healthy foods you could ever eat. Fish are like swimming vitamin

supplements. Their high oil content is both healthier for you and easier for your body to digest (especially when compared to the fatty oils found in beef, pork, and other red meats). Eating more fish will help prevent all kinds of age related illnesses from dementia to wrinkling skin. Try to eat 3 to 4 servings of fish per week minimum (note: one serving is about 4 ounces). You will have to be careful of mercury content. Not all fish contain dangerous levels of mercury and it's not dangerous to eat some high mercury fish sometimes. But try to limit yourself to low mercury fish and only occasionally eat the high mercury ones. The fish with the highest mercury content include swordfish, shark, king mackerel, and tilefish. Fish with low mercury content include snapper, lobster, light tuna, trout, crab, oysters, salmon, tilapia, anchovies, and herring (among others).

4. **Chocolate:** yes, chocolate is a super food! Dieting never sounded so delicious before, did it? Chocolate is rich in antioxidants and flavanols. These are

responsible for preserving your blood vessels so that they stay strong. Healthy blood vessels can reduce your blood pressure, decrease your risk for diabetes and prevent both kidney disease and dementia. Healthy blood vessels also ensure that you have healthy blood circulation which is necessary to give your skin a youthful and lively appearance. It can also decrease your risk for heart attack and stroke by nearly 40%. The important thing to note here is that you need to eat *dark* chocolate to get these benefits. Milk chocolate is far too diluted. It does not contain enough actual chocolate for you to get these benefits. To be considered dark chocolate, it needs to contain at least 70% cocoa. Avoid the kinds that have fillings like peanut butter as these often contain hydrogenated oils which are terrible for your body. To get the full benefits, all you need to eat is one piece of dark chocolate per day (about the size of a single square or a Hershey's kiss). But, hey, this is your health we are talking about: there's no reason you shouldn't eat a whole bar of dark chocolate each day!

5. **Nuts:** nuts are tiny age fighting soldiers that happen to make delicious snacks. Nuts like walnuts, almonds, pecans, or cashews (*not* peanuts) will lower your cholesterol, improve your metabolism, and strengthen your immune system. They also help you to lower your calorie intake so that you can lose some weight. This is because, even though nuts are high in calories, they keep you feeling full longer so that you eat less junk food. If you are craving unhealthy salty foods, eating a small snack of nuts instead will eliminate that craving and give you a healthy, long-lasting boost of energy. They also contain high levels of vitamin E which rejuvenates your skin tissue. The high oil content helps your skin in much the same way as olive oil. Plus, studies show that people who eat nuts can even increase their life span! So eat nuts every single day and you can start looking younger *and* live longer!

6. **Wine:** specifically *red* wine has been proven in study after study to be amazing for your health. That

doesn't mean you should be downing two or three bottles per day. One glass in the evening should suffice. But don't feel bad if you polish off a bottle or two in one night with some friends every once in awhile. Red wine contains something called "reservatrol" which is a high power antioxidant that protects your arteries and prevents inflammation. It also prevents your cells from dying prematurely and keeps them healthy, young and able to reproduce themselves without mutations or defects.

7. **Blueberries:** blueberries get their vibrant color from something called anthocyanin. Anthocynanin is an anti-inflammatory antioxidant that helps preserve the brain and skin. Eating about 1 cup of blueberries per day will not only prevent age related mental illnesses like Alzheimer's or dementia but will actually improve your cognitive skills right now by as much as 5%. They are also a great source of vitamin E which (as you have read about nuts and olive oil) is one of the most important vitamins for keeping your skin looking young, healthy and wrinkle free. If that

wasn't enough, the vitamins and antioxidants found in blueberries also protect our DNA from damage to keep your body younger even at the genetic level.

8. **Strawberries:** strawberries contain many of the same properties as blueberries. Although, blueberries are admittedly the stronger berry. They contain more of the good stuff than strawberries do. Regardless, strawberries are a great super food to keep you looking and feeling younger. They also pack a high dosage of vitamin C which is essential for maintaining a strong immune system. With a strong immune system, you can fight off illnesses better. The less often you become sick, the less damage your cells have to suffer. The flu and common cold may not be deadly but they can have long lasting effects on your body. If you find yourself getting sick often, your body will start aging before its time. So it is extremely important to maintain a strong immune system.

9. **Tomatoes:** we all know tomatoes are healthy but it rarely gets included in lists of super foods. But

tomatoes actually have a lot of hidden properties most people don't know about. Recently, scientists have discovered the cancer preventing powers of lycopene (found in tomatoes). Lycopene is a kind of carotenoid (vitamin A). Studies have proven that eating a diet high in lycopene will protect your skin from sun damage. Sun damage is one of the biggest environmental causes of wrinkled skin. In fact, eating enough lycopene on daily basis has been shown to decrease sun damage by as much as 33%. To get the highest concentrations of lycopene, eat more tomato paste rather than actual tomatoes. For the full benefits of lycopene, eat at least 5 tablespoons of tomato paste daily. You can add this to a pasta dish or simply mix it with olive oil and herbs to use as a dip for carrots or other fresh veggies.

10. **Tofu:** soy products like tofu, soy milk or just plain soybeans (often referred to as "edamame") slow down the deterioration of collagen and elastin. Collagen and elastin are the main components of your skin that keep it firm, soft, and radiant. Soy

products contain isoflavones. These are powerful antioxidants that can protect your collagen and elastin from damage. Studies have found that isoflavones promote elastin production and prevent elastin deterioration. Plus, tofu (like yogurt) serves as a great base for a wide number of dishes. This kind of versatility will ensure that you never have to get bored of eating healthy and looking younger!

11. Coffee: like red wine, coffee contains powerful antioxidants like reservatrol that help strengthen your blood vessels and improve circulation. So if you are not much of wine drinker, coffee will make a great alternative. Be sure to practice moderation, though. One cup of coffee per day will give you the full anti-aging benefits. Try to keep your coffee intake down to 1 or 2 cups per day. The best way to drink your coffee (for health reasons) is to drink it black. Most people find the flavor too strong, though. If you take your coffee with milk, that's fine. But you should absolutely cut out all sugar. Adding whole milk (or even half and half) will usually add enough sweetness to tone down the strong flavor of coffee. Milk contains lactose which is a kind of sugar. It may take a couple of days to get used to but soon you will learn to appreciate the flavor of coffee without sugar. If you want to go a step further, slowly decrease the amount of milk or cream you add to your coffee each day until you are able to tolerate (and even enjoy) the strong flavor of black coffee.

12. **Beans:** research has started to come out that proves beans are a magical fruit for more reasons than you thought. They are high in fiber which is essential to a healthy digestive system. A high fiber diet (meaning between 30-40 grams of fiber per day) will keep your digestive system clean and decrease the amount of toxins in your body. Fewer toxins in the body means less risk for premature or accelerated aging. In addition to being high in fiber, they are high in protein. Proteins are the building blocks of your cells. If you aren't getting enough protein, your cells won't be able to develop healthily. This can lead to premature aging and other age related problems.

Beans are also rich in antioxidants which will fight off the toxins already in your body (all while the fiber is flushing out the toxins in your food before they can enter your blood). If reading all that hasn't already made you get up and go grab a can of beans; you should know that they are also high in iron, vitamin B and many other important vitamins and minerals that keep you energized and youthful.

13. **Garlic:** garlic is a pungent little powerhouse of anti-aging compounds. It's great for your heart, your brain, your skin, your digestive system, your immune system and just about everything else. It is essentially a whole body system restorer. It has powerful antioxidants and even acts as an antibacterial that targets the bad bacteria and toxins in your body. It also helps your circulation so that your skin will look more radiant and you will feel more energized and youthful. It also helps you resist common illnesses like the cold. It also slows down cellular decay, diminishes cellulite, and repairs damaged skin. Try to

eat 2 to 3 cloves of garlic per day so that you can get the full range of benefits.

14.**Avocado:** if you aren't already in love with these delicious fruits; it's time to make avocados a major part of your daily routine. Avocados contain high amounts of vitamin E, healthy plant oils, antioxidants, vitamin B, folic acid, potassium, and much, much more. All of these help combat the aging process by lowering cholesterol, lowering blood pressure, making your skin suppler, and strengthening your bones. Eat it straight out of the shell with a spoon; puree it into a guacamole dip; or chop it up into your salad. There are millions of ways to eat avocadoes and all of them are delicious (and work to combat aging).

15.**Whole Grains:** whole grains are high in fiber as well as vitamins and minerals. They also contain a lot of powerful antioxidants that help improve circulation which decreases the aging process of your internal organs while making your skin appear more radiant.

An important thing to remember, though, is that whole grains are *not* the same as whole wheat. Breads and other products that claim to be "whole wheat" are misleadingly marketed and do not actually contain whole *grains*. You want to look for products that specifically say whole grain because many of these health benefits come from the germ of the grain. During the process of making white breads and whole wheat breads, this germ is removed from the grain completely. So you will *not* be getting any of the amazing benefits of whole grains by eating whole wheat products. You need to make sure it is specifically labeled as whole *grain.*

Eating Habits that Slow Down Aging

1. **Eat Breakfast:** scientists have been realizing more and more just how important it is to eat a healthy breakfast every morning. It jump starts your metabolism, provides your body with a stable source of energy and reduces your risk for all sorts of age related problems (mental

deterioration and physical deterioration). Start each day with a complete balanced breakfast: high fiber, high protein, and high nutrient. If you (like most of us) don't have the time in the morning to cook a big nutritious diet, try out some smoothie recipes. Carrots, bananas, berries, green leafy vegetables and tofu make great foods to throw in a blender. Add in some yogurt, milk and honey to make a sweet, creamy treat that will fuel you for the rest of the day. You can also throw in some sliced almonds or other nuts at the end for a nice crunchy texture that also adds an extra boost of protein (and healthy plant fats!) Have fun with your smoothies. Experiment with different combinations and write down the recipes for the ones you like best. They are quick, delicious, and make it much easier to guarantee that you are eating enough nutritious foods.

2. **Drink Water:** as much as 75% of Americans are living in a state of chronic dehydration. This is because we tend to drink soda, coffee, and other beverages that *feel* like they are hydrating but are actually *de*hydrating us. To make it worse, we don't balance this out by drinking enough water. If you walk away from this book with just

one lesson, let it be that you need to drink more water. The bare *minimum* should be about 2 liters per day. Going up to three liters a day for the first few weeks will help you recover from chronic dehydration and reverse its negative effects. Chronic dehydration causes joint problems, chronic fatigue, and speeds up the process of aging. This is because water is an absolute essential to keep our body running smoothly. Chronic dehydration is like driving a car without oil. Without oil, your car's engine parts will dry out, rub against each other causing friction, overheating, and making all the different parts become brittle and fragile. The same thing happens to your body. When you are dehydrated, your cells don't have the fluid they need to function normally. Your muscles will begin to break down, your organs will start to fail and your skin will dry out and lose its vibrancy. If you aren't already in the habit of drinking 2 to 3 liters of water per day, buy a reusable water bottle and start carrying it in your purse everywhere you go. Instead of having soda or juice with your lunch, have water. Instead of just drinking a cup of coffee in the morning. Have a glass of water with your coffee.

3. **Stop Yo-yo Dieting:** fad diets come and go. And many people will jump on the band wagon, dieting heavily for a few weeks or a few months before giving up and going back to their old unhealthy eating habits. This "yo-yoing" between diets wreaks havoc on your body and can cause actually cause you to age faster than usual. Instead, just strive to always eat a healthy, balanced diet with plenty of vegetables and other nutritious foods. Sticking to a balanced and nutritious diet will help you maintain a healthy, youthful appearance well into your later years. This is because your body will be consistently fed all the nutrients it needs to maintain a healthy, strong system in every possible aspect. A strong, healthy internal body means a strong, youthful external appearance. Yo-yo dieting (especially when you go on extreme diets like fasts) will leave you looking grey, aged, and tired. Your skin won't have that youthful glow that comes with a nutritious diet.

4. **Embrace Fatty Foods:** I know, you just read earlier in this chapter that you need to cut down on the fatty meats. But that is specifically in reference to meat. Your body is not built to digest an exclusively meat diet. You

are not a carnivore. Fatty plant foods (avocados, olive oil, and so on) are much easier for your body to break down and are extremely healthy for you. Studies have actually found that high (plant) fat diets can actually help you *lose* weight. It is also amazing for your skin. Plant fats help increase the elasticity of your skin and give it a healthy, youthful glow. Plus, when companies manufacture "low fat" foods, they usually replace the fat with refined sugar to make up for the loss of favor. That means that they are taking out the healthy fat you *should* be eating and replacing it with unhealthy refined sugar that you should actually be *avoiding.* Fatty foods also keep you feeling fuller longer because the fat is more satisfying and takes a little longer to digest than simple sugars. This keeps your blood sugar levels stabilized so you don't experience those sudden bursts of energy followed by fatigue and sluggishness.

5. **Stop Depending on Supplements:** supplements can be helpful for those who have medical deficiencies in certain vitamins or minerals but you should not use them as a *substitute* for healthy, nutritious food. It is so much better to get your vitamins and minerals from

actual food sources rather than swallowing a pill. Plus, taking supplements on a daily basis if you don't have a medical deficiency can actually increase your risk for overdosing on those vitamins. Overdoses can cause just as many problems as deficiencies for some vitamins. There is also the risk that if you depend on a supplement for nutrition, you will trick yourself into believing that it is ok to fill your body with junk food since you already got all your vitamins from your morning supplement. Filling your body with junk (like the foods mentioned earlier in this chapter) will cause you to age faster than normal even though you are taking a vitamin supplement. So instead of a daily supplement every morning, opt for a delicious (and nutritious) morning breakfast to get your day started. That's a lot more tasty than swallowing a giant vitamin supplement, anyway.

6. **Make Your Own Salad Dressing:** premade salad dressings are filled with preservatives and excess salt and sugar. They also often contain unhealthy forms of fat that your body cannot easily digest. Making your own salad dressing is surprisingly easy and guarantees that you have a fresh, healthy, and delicious dressing for

your salads. Fresh lime or lemon juice with olive oil, herbs, and seasonings will actually add nutrition (as well as *healthy* fat) to your salad rather than decrease the nutrition value like premade dressings do. Plus, you can tailor the recipe to your exact tastes so it will be even more delicious than the store bought kind *and* you won't have to feel the slightest amount of guilt for pouring on the dressing.

7. **Practice Balance:** you do not have to cut out all your favorite foods completely just for the sake of looking younger. You just need to practice balance. Make sure that you are eating mostly healthy foods from the list of super foods that slow or reverse aging and moderate the amount of foods you eat from the list of foods that speed up aging. If you take care to give your body all the nutrients it needs to stay healthy; it will be much stronger and much more capable of dealing with the unhealthy foods without suffering their negative effects. With that in mind, however, you should probably try to cut out refined sugar entirely. There are a lot of healthier substitutes out there like honey and natural sweeteners. Avoid artificial sweeteners, though. These

can be just as dangerous (and sometimes *more* dangerous) than the refined sugar that it is meant to replace.

Eating a healthy, nutritious diet provides your body with the building blocks it needs to repair the damage already caused by aging and prevent damage from occurring in the future. However, your diet is just one half of the story. If you want to look younger and more radiant; you also need to get active and start exercising. You'll learn some practical tips for making exercise a part of your regular routine in the next chapter.

Chapter 3: Exercise Your Way to Youth

Exercise keeps your body in peak physical condition so that your muscles, bones, and inner workings stay young and healthy. As you have already read earlier in this book: the best way to have a younger looking outside is to make sure you have a younger feeling inside.

The best thing about exercise is that it is all good for you. There are thousands of different ways to be active so you can choose whatever activity or sport you enjoy the most. The most important thing is that you are having fun and elevating your heart rate for at least 20 minutes per day.

The purpose of this chapter is not to tell you exactly how you have to exercise in order to look younger. It's just here to help you get inspired and give you some ideas in case you aren't really sure where to start.

Yoga

Yoga is a great workout to help prevent aging. Not only does it improve circulation, it strengthens your bones and muscles and gives you more flexibility. This will give you better posture which will take years off your appearance. It will also firm and tone your muscles so that you don't have to worry about any jiggle or sagging.

There are a lot of great yoga courses out there for all experience levels. You can get a video to do yoga from home or you can sign up for a class at your local gym or recreational center. Some of the best anti aging yoga poses are the following:

1. Standing Forward Bend

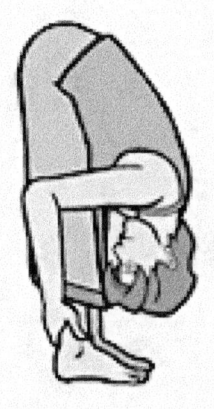

2. Proud Warrior

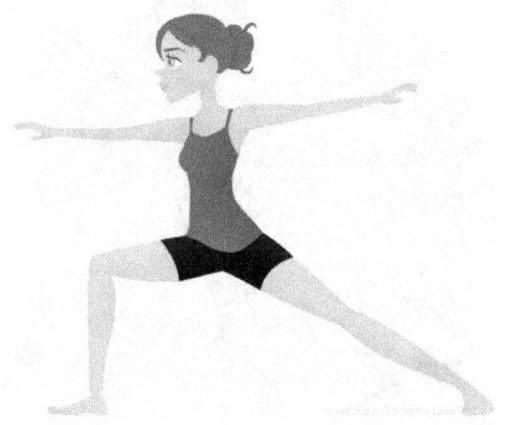

3. Side Stretch

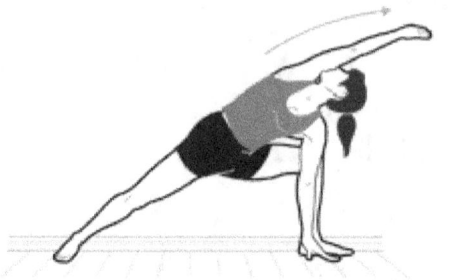

4. Tree Pose

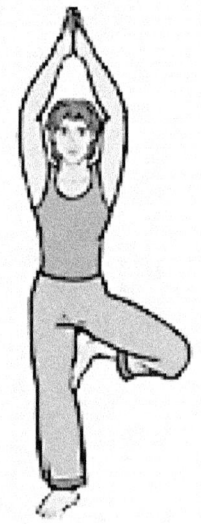

5. Upward Facing Dog

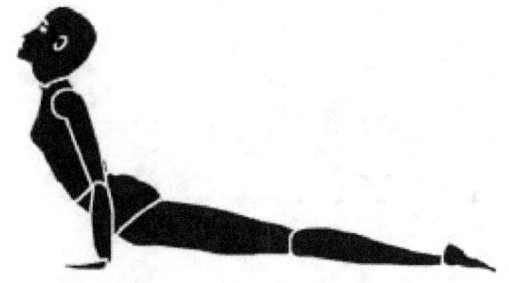

6. Seated Twist

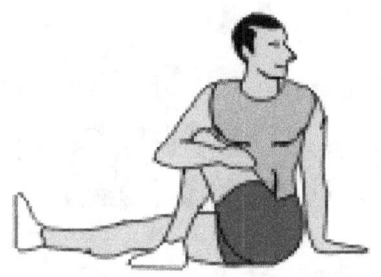

7. Bridge Pose

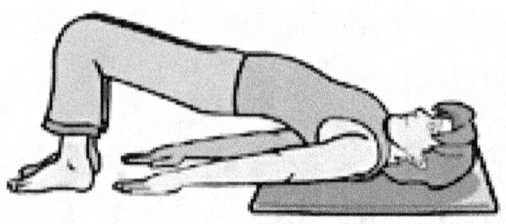

8. Reclining Twist

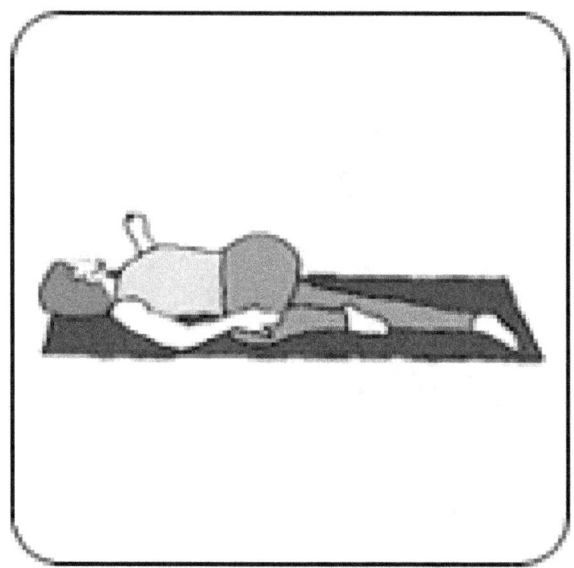

These are just a few of hundreds of possible poses in yoga. If you are a beginner, you will want to start with the simpler poses and possibly buy some of the equipment like blocks, straps and pillows that help you do the pose fully without overstraining your muscles. As you increase your strength and flexibility, you can stop using the extra equipment.

Doing yoga on a daily basis can help reduce cellulite and firm the skin. It will keep you looking younger and it is extremely healthy for you. It also has countless proven benefits for your mental and emotional state. So yoga is a great all around treatment that can make you younger in every possible way.

Cardio

Cardiovascular exercise is any exercise that gets your blood pumping. This includes walking, running, swimming, hiking, biking, and other activities where you can feel your heart start to race. Cardio exercises are a great way to look younger because they improve circulation which keeps your skin looking radiant and alive.

It also makes you feel younger on every level. You feel more energized, in shape, and ready to take on anything. This will give you a lively and youthful expression as you take on your day. If you are currently pretty inactive (i.e. – you don't make a conscious effort to exercise) then you want to make sure you start out slowly. For example, you can follow this plan:

	Week 1	Week 2	Week 3	Week 4
Day 1	Walk 20 Minutes	Run 5 Minutes Walk 25 Minutes	Rest	Walk 5 Minutes Run 15 Minutes Walk 10 Minutes
Day 2	Walk 20 Minutes	Rest	Run 10 Minutes Walk 5 Minutes Run 10 Minutes Walk 10 Minutes	Walk 5 Minutes Run 15 Minutes Walk 10 Minutes
Day 3	Rest	Run 5 Minutes Walk 25 Minutes	Run 10 Minutes Walk 5 Minutes Run 10 Minutes Walk 10 Minutes	Rest
Day 4	Walk 30 Minutes	Run 5 Minutes Walk 15 Minutes Run 5 Minutes Walk 5	Rest	Walk 5 Minutes Run 15 Minutes Walk 10 Minutes

		Minutes		
Day 5	Walk 30 Minutes	Rest	Walk 5 Minutes Run 10 Minutes Walk 5 Minutes Run 10 Minutes Walk 5 Minutes	Walk 5 Minutes Run 20 Minutes Walk 10 Minutes
Day 6	Rest	Run 10 Minutes Walk 10 Minutes Run 5 Minutes Walk 5 Minutes	Walk 5 Minutes Run 10 Minutes Walk 5 Minutes Run 10 Minutes Walk 5 Minutes	Rest
Day 7	Walk 30 Minutes	Run 10 Minutes Walk 10 Minutes Run 5 Minutes Walk 5 Minutes	Rest	Walk 5 Minutes Run 20 Minutes Walk 10 Minutes

If this schedule is moving too fast for you and you feel that you aren't ready to increase the intensity when the schedule suggests it; then continue at the pace you are comfortable with. This plan is intended as a guideline to show you how you can go from not exercising at all to running 20 minutes a day.

You'll notice that there are some days where you are supposed to rest. It is important to give your body time to recover. The best exercise schedule is 2 days on, 1 day off. That is how this one has been set up.

Strength Exercises

Strength exercises are those exercises that focus on building muscle rather than speed, endurance, flexibility or agility. These are exercises like weight lifting, squats, or pushups. If you don't have a weight training set at home and don't want to go to the gym to lift weights alongside dozens of beefed up guys; there are some great strength exercises you can do at home using just your own body weight and common household items.

Strength exercises are an excellent way to get rid of cellulite and tone your body. Doing strength training doesn't necessarily mean you have to become a bulked up body builder. You can use them simply to tone and shape your body so that there is no cellulite, excess jiggling, or sagging skin. Here are some good strength exercises you can do at home without needing any other equipment:

1. Push Ups

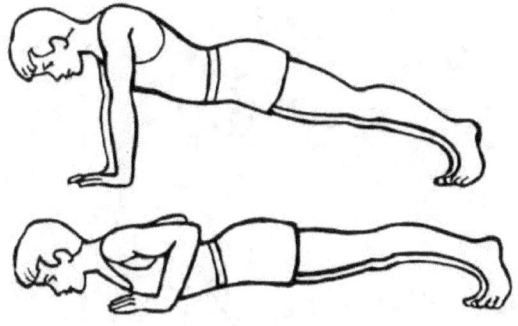

2. Squats

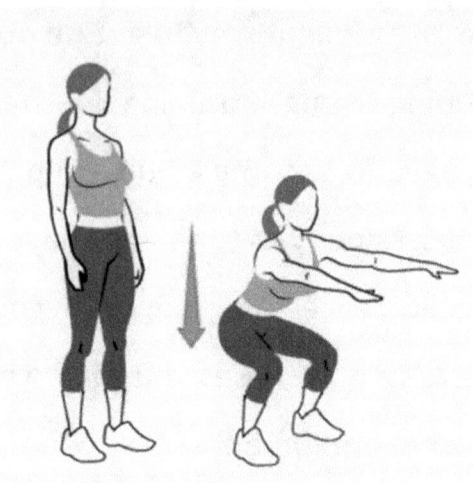

3. Lunges

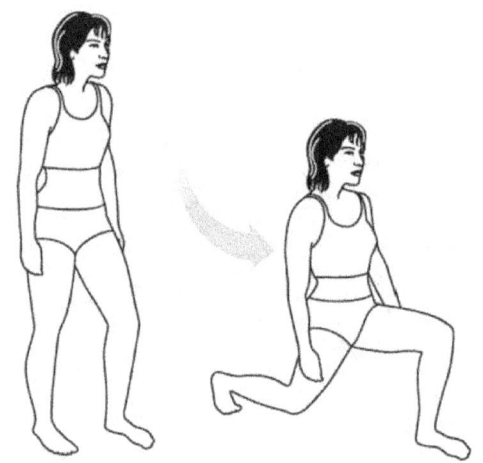

4. Triceps Dips

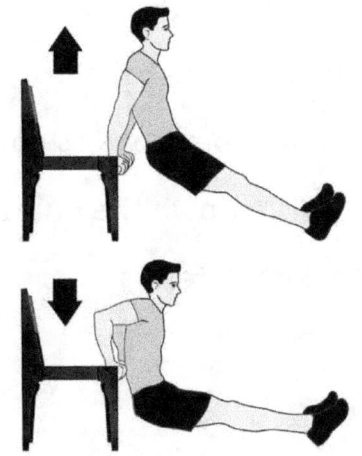

5. Dynamic Prone Plank

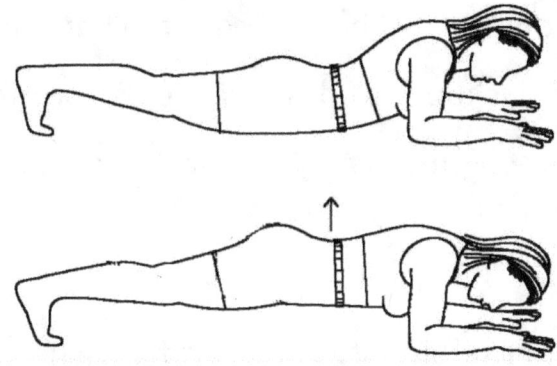

6. Crunches

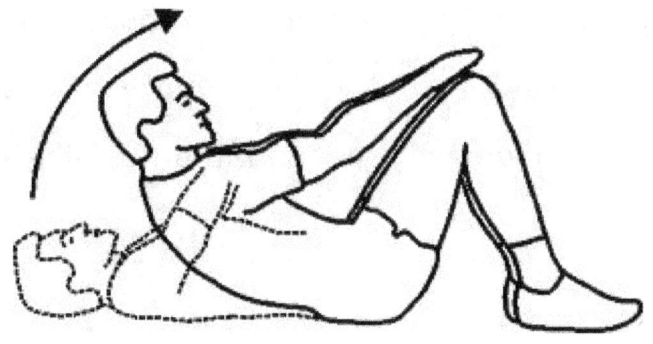

There is no magic number for how many repetitions of these exercises to do. The best rule of thumb to follow is this: the first day of exercise, do as many repetitions as you can without overstraining your muscles. Write down the number of repetitions you were able to complete.

Do not include any half repetitions, only include the number you were able to complete fully. For example, if you were doing pushups, only count the number of full pushups you completed. One pushup is a full sequence of lowering down to the ground and then pushing all the way back up again.

Then, each day of exercise after that, add anywhere from 1 to 5 more repetitions to that original number that you did on the first day. Continue adding repetitions until you feel you have reached the shape and fitness level that you want to achieve. Then, maintain that workout pattern without adding any new repetitions.

Remember to include one day of rest for every two days of exercise. This is especially important with strength exercises because your muscle needs time to repair itself and grow.

Sports

Sports are a great way to get active and get enough exercise in your regular routine. You can do team sports or individual sports. Team sports have the added benefit of keeping you motivated because you are part of a team. Individual sports, on the other hand, are better for those who prefer to go at their own pace.

Whatever type of sport you choose; you will usually get a great combination of cardio and strength training. Some great sports for staying young include soccer, tennis, swimming, biking, and golf. Swimming is especially great for those who have weak joints or arthritis because it is low impact on the joints while still providing a great cardio workout and even building up muscular strength (which could ultimately even help your joints!)

Facial Exercises

In addition to physical exercises that get your body looking younger, you should also do some facial exercises that keep the skin on your face and neck firm and wrinkle free. This will make sure that your face looks as young as your body. Here are five exercises you can do to help reduce wrinkles and improve circulation to the skin on your face. Do these daily to have radiant, glowing wrinkle free skin:

1. The V massage

   This is meant to help reduce crow's feet, puffiness, and raise drooping eyelids. To do it, make a V or peace sign with both hands. Press the middle finger into the corner of your eyebrow at the top of your nose. Press the index finger on your temple at the other end of your eyebrow. Apply a fair amount of pressure to each of these points. Look up toward the ceiling and raise your lower lids like you are squinting up at something. Repeat this 6 times and then shut your eyes tightly for 10 seconds.

2. The Smile Shaper

   This exercise is to help improve the cheek lines and reduce sagging skin. Start by pulling your lips inward tightly to cover your teeth. You should be making an O shape with your mouth. While doing this, smile as widely as you can without moving your lips away from your teeth. Repeat this 6 times. On the sixth time, hold the smile, tilt your head back and press your index finger on the center of your chin. Push your jaw up and down with your finger (while holding the smile you have been holding). Do this 6 times. Then relax.

3. The Forehead Massage

   The forehead massage is good for minimizing the horizontal wrinkles that appear on the forehead. To do this exercise, place both hands on your forehead with the fingers of each hand meeting each other at the center of your forehead. Make sure the fingers are spread so that the index is at the base of your hairline and the pinky is just above your eyebrows. Gently sweep the fingers outward (toward your temples) while applying light pressure in order to tighten the skin and smooth out the wrinkles. Repeat this 10 times.

4. The Under Eye Lift

    This exercise is good for drooping eye brows and to reduce the appearance of sunken in eyebrows. Begin by pulling your lips inward to cover your teeth as you did with the smile smoother exercise above. Make an O shape with your mouth again. But do not smile. Then, place your index fingers on your lower eyelids (so that your fingers are pointing toward your nose). Move the fingers downward, pressing lightly so as to pull your lower eyelids down with them. Now, look upward at the ceiling and flutter your upper eyelids while still holding your lower eyelids down with your fingers. Do this continuously for 30 seconds.

5. The Neck Smoother

This one is meant for the loose skin and wrinkles that often form on the neck with age. Keeping your neck smooth and wrinkle free will take years of your appearance because this is one of the key areas that reveal your age. To do this exercise, begin sitting up straight with your shoulders back. Look straight ahead. Place your finger tips at the bottom of your neck, just above your collar bone. Press your fingers into your neck gently (don't choke yourself!) Now, fully extend your neck by tilting your head back and looking upward toward the ceiling. Gently massage the skin of the neck downward toward your collar bone as you keep your head tilted back. Do this for 10 seconds. Then bring the head all the way down to the chest. Repeat this sequence three times. On the third time, as you pull the skin downward with your fingers, hold it instead of massaging and take four deep, slow breaths.

General Exercise Tips

Exercise is an extremely important part of keeping your youthful appearance. Between proper diet (which you learned about in chapter 2) and adequate exercise (which you have just now read about), you can take decades off your appearance. This is because unlike the lotions, surgeries, and other anti aging methods out there, diet and exercise fight aging at the cellular level so that you don't just look younger, you actually *are* physically younger (in the sense that your body is not aging as fast as it was).

So to help you ensure that you get enough exercise, here are a few extra tips for exercising:

- Explore: whether you already have a set workout routine you have been doing or you have never worked out a day in your life; the important thing is to try out a lot of different kinds of exercise before you settle on any. This helps you stay motivated because you find a form of exercise that you genuinely enjoy so that you will look forward to getting out doing it.

- Variety is the spice of life: even when you find one type of exercise you enjoy, don't feel like you have to just stick to that one. As you do that one regularly, make sure you try out other ones here and there as well. Spice up your routine by having a few different types of exercise that you do regularly. For example, you can alternate between doing strength training, yoga, and running. Having variety will make sure that you never get bored with your routine.

- Track your progress: keep a daily log of the exercise you do (and even the food you eat). Even if you don't have a specific goal weight or shape you are trying to achieve and just want to keep yourself looking younger, tracking your progress is a great way to stay motivated. You can see how much you have improved since your first workout. This is a huge motivator for those days when you feel like you have sort of stagnated.

- Know your body: above all, listen to what your body is telling you. If you are overdoing it on the exercise, you could end up causing serious damage that could leave you bed ridden for months. That's months of not being able to exercise so you will risk falling out of shape again. So if you feel like you have hit your limit, don't try to push yourself past it. The more you exercise, the better you will get. Allow your body to improve at its own rate.

- Exercise with friends or sign up for a class: a great way to stay motivated to exercise regularly is to do it with others. Find a workout buddy or sign up for a training class at your local gym or recreational center. Having others that you workout with will help you get off your butt on those days when you don't feel especially motivated to exercise.

Now that you have read through these first three chapters, you are actually completely ready to start reducing and reversing the signs of aging! The next three chapters will provide you with additional tips for looking younger. These tips do not actually target the seven causes of aging that you read about in chapter 1. Instead, they are more focused on external methods of reducing the signs of aging such as dressing younger.

In the next chapter (chapter 4) you will learn about some home remedies that can help reduce the signs of aging. These are skin treatments that you can make using everyday ingredients from your kitchen.

Chapter 4: Reverse the Aging Process with Home Remedies

In this chapter, you will learn about recipes for face masks and skin treatments that you can make at home using everyday ingredients from your kitchen. These home remedies are not meant to be used by themselves and won't complete erase the signs of aging by themselves. Instead, you should use them in combination with diet and exercise.

After the first few treatments, you will already begin to notice some reduction of wrinkles, cellulite, and other signs of aging on the skin. But, as mentioned earlier, to complete erase these signs, you should follow the diet and exercise tips you have read about in chapters 2 and 3.

Coffee Body Scrub

This one is really simple and surprisingly effective. While in the shower, mix ¼ cup coffee grounds with the hot water from your shower. Massage this into your skin for about 10 minutes. Stand away from the shower stream so that the coffee does not get immediately rinsed away as you are scrubbing. Do this twice per week for 10 minutes each time. The coffee grounds improve your circulation and tightens your skin. You will notice somewhat tighter skin almost immediately but allow about 4 weeks for dramatic results.

Cayenne Lemon Elixir

Mix juice from one lemon and one teaspoon cayenne pepper in 4 ounces of warm (but not hot) water. Drink this mixture 3 times daily. Within 30 days, you will notice your skin become significantly firmer and will feel better overall as this is also a great way to detoxify your body and boost your energy levels.

Olive Juniper Massage

Combine about 20 drops of Juniper essential oil with a ½ cup of olive oil. Massage this all over your skin. Spend extra time massaging it into the problematic areas such as thighs, neck, and upper arms. Your skin will immediately become smoother and after about 3 to 4 weeks, you will begin to notice visibly firmer skin and a significant reduction to cellulite and wrinkles.

Coconut Brush

This is one of the most effective home remedy treatments for cellulite and also firms and moisturizes your skin in general. Smooth coconut oil over your entire body (if you get pure coconut oil with no additives, it is completely safe for all areas, including the face). Then, take a dry brush to massage the problem areas (focusing on cellulite and wrinkles). Immediately after the treatment, your skin will feel sensitive and there may be some redness but this effect wears off quickly and if you do this daily, your cellulite will be almost completely gone after just 30 days. Your skin will also be smoother, firmer, and more radiant as a result of this treatment. Note: while you can use the coconut oil safely on your face, do not use the dry brush on your face as the skin there is too sensitive for this part of the treatment. Instead, just spend about 10 minutes gently massaging the coconut oil into your face. You can use the facial exercise techniques you learned about in chapter 3 with the coconut oil to further reduce wrinkling around the eyes, mouth, neck, and forehead.

Lemon Rinse

This one is an extremely easy way to erase liver spots and even out your skin tone. Simply squeeze the juice from a lemon on the areas of your skin with liver spots or other blemishes you want to erase. Lightly rub it into the area and let sit for about 15 minutes. Then, rinse it off with water. Do this once per day. Your skin tone will even out and liver spots will begin to noticeably disappear after about 2-3 weeks of daily treatments.

Lemon Cream Mask

This mask will even out your skin tone as well as reduce wrinkles and firm the skin on your face. To make it, combine 1 teaspoon freshly squeezed lemon juice, ½ teaspoon of milk cream, and 1 teaspoon of egg whites. Mix well and gently spread across your face and neck. Let it sit for 15 minutes.

Then, rinse it off with cold water and gently pat the skin dry with a soft towel.

Cucumber Curd Mask

Combine a ½ cup of milk curds with 2 teaspoons of finely grated cucumber. Apply the mixture to your face and neck area and let sit for 20 minutes. Make sure you apply the mixture to the under eye area as well because it is extremely effective for bags and dark circles. Rinse with cold water and pat the skin dry gently with a soft towel. Do this twice per week and your skin will become firmer and brighter.

White Tea Facial

This one is great for the bags under the eyes as well as reducing the appearance of wrinkles on the rest of your face. To do this, start by heating water on the stove. Do not let it boil. Instead, heat it just until it is hot to the touch. Test this by dipping your finger into the water. As soon as it is too hot to leave your finger in the water, it is ready. You do not want to let the water get too hot because it will destroy the chemical structure of the tea and prevent it from being an effective treatment. Pour the water over the white tea bag in a cup. Let steep for about 10 minutes. Then dip a soft washcloth into the tea and place it on your face. Be sure that it is pressed down onto your eye area as well. Leave the warm, tea soaked cloth on your face for about 10 minutes. You can do this nightly before bed since it also happens to be very relaxing and soothing.

Chapter 5: Freshen Up Your Wardrobe and Look Younger

In this chapter you will learn a few quick fashion tips so that you can dress younger. Many people try to dress younger in order to give themselves a more youthful appearance. However, dressing like a 15 year old when you are in your 40s or 50s is not going to make you look younger. It's going to make you look ridiculous.

That's why the tips you will read here go beyond just shopping in the teen section of the clothing store. Instead, you will get practical tips for dressing in a way that makes you appear younger but in a more natural way (i.e. – it doesn't look so obvious that you are trying to dress younger).

1. **Nude tights:** nude tights should be a staple item of your wardrobe now, preferably with a control top. They do wonders for your legs from gently shaping

them to evening the skin tone and disguising cellulite, wrinkles, or liver spots.

2. **Just above the knee skirts:** to look more youthful, ditch the long skirts that go below the knee (except for your floor length gowns). Above the knee skirts will freshen up your look and give you a youthful appearance. But be careful, you shouldn't be wearing miniskirts. Skirts should end right above the knee so that you look youthful without looking like you are trying to pass for 15. A good rule of thumb: if you can't bend over in it without exposing your underwear, don't wear it.

3. **Know your body type:** not every trend suits every body type. Know what sort of patterns, colors, and cuts look the most flattering on your and stick with those rather than just buying whatever is currently in vogue. For example, if you are a little on the bustier side, avoid V necks or very low cut tops as these will sit awkwardly on your chest. On the other hand, if you have a smaller chest, go for the lower cut tops and skip the high necklines.

4. **Embrace color:** we all know the little black dress is an essential. But once your over 40, a colorful dress can actually do you a lot more favors. A bright (but still flattering for your skin tone) color will brighten your look and make you look younger and fresher. Remember not to go too short, though.

5. **No more ruffles:** frills, ruffles and other textures on clothing look adorable on children but awkward on older women. You want to try to dress more youthful while still maintaining your natural elegance. Try to stick with fitted shapes: fitted pants, fitted blazers, straight leg jeans. You can have flowing dresses but avoid anything with poof, ruffle, or frill.

6. **Wear white:** white is a wonderful color that will brighten you up while still looking beautifully elegant. Every woman should own a white button down blouse that flatters her figure. You should also have a white skirt, white dress, white blazer, and so on. But remember not to dress head to toe in white. If you were the white blouse, wear a darker skirt or pant. If you wear the white blazer, wear a darker blouse.

Combine however you want, just make sure you let the white item really pop.

7. **Don't overdo it:** hair, makeup, and clothing should be relatively simple. You want to accentuate natural beauty. If you put on bright blue eye shadow, you won't look younger, you'll just call more attention to any crow's feet or wrinkles around the eyes. Instead, stick with more neutral tones when it comes to make up. If you want to add a splash of color, use accessories. But remember, if you wear colorful accessories, make sure your outfit is a neutral color (whites, blacks, and tans) so that the colorful accessories pop rather than disappearing into the outfit.

Final Word

Now that you have finished this book, you are ready to start looking and feeling younger from the inside out. You can use any of these strategies you liked best but keep in mind: for the best results, you should use a combination of them all.

By eating right, exercising regularly, and dressing yourself more youthfully, you will soon be looking decades younger and (more importantly) *feeling* that much younger too! Plus, now that you have a basic understanding of the 7 causes of aging, you will be better able to tell which anti-aging methods will work and which ones are totally bunk.

In fact, by using the methods mentioned in this book, you can save thousands on expensive surgeries and lotions designed to make you look younger. These expensive treatments may have temporary effects but if you want lasting results, use the methods in this book.

Now get out there and let your youthful spirit shine!

www.ingramcontent.com/pod-product-compliance
Lightning Source LLC
Chambersburg PA
CBHW070402290526
45790CB00004B/1597